DR BARBARA NUTRITIONAL GUIDE FOR BREAST CANCER

The Ultimate Guide on How to Stop and Degenerate Cancer Cells of the Breast Through Dr Barbara O'Neill Alkaline Plant-Based Diet

KATHONA BODI

ISBN: 9798333286086

CONTENTS

Introduction

Recent reports show that, in the United States, at least 1 in every 8 women will suffer from breast cancer in their lifetime. If you do the math, that's around 13% of the total female population.

In fact, breast cancer is currently the second most common type of cancer women suffer. This shows how serious the disease is and encourages the need to create more awareness among women.

Just like any other cancer disease, diet is thought to be partly responsible for breast cancer. Other causes may be linked to lifestyle choices, reproductive history, age, and other factors. In essence, you can greatly reduce your risk of getting the disease if you make good dietary choices. Likewise, for people already diagnosed with the condition, changing your diet can be an effective way to manage symptoms and aid your recovery in the long run.

Just to give you an idea, foods rich in fat can cause obesity, which can increase your risk of getting breast cancer. On the other hand, following a plant-based diet can greatly reduce your risk of getting the disease or managing the symptoms.

The Dr Barbara Diet is a plant-based vegan diet which can be effective in supporting cancer patients and aiding recovery. Besides eating healthy, one of the best things you can also do as a cancer patient is fast. Fasting can accelerate your healing when done properly and in combination with the right diet. This book will show you how to effectively incorporate both in your treatment.

What Is Breast Cancer?

Breast cancer is a type of cancer that occurs when the breast cells mutate and grow out of control to form tumors. This can happen in one or both breasts. One of the main dangers of breast cancer is that when untreated, the tumors can multiply and spread throughout the body leading to a fatal situation.

The most affected group of breast cancer seems to be women, usually above the age of 50. The disease can also affect men and younger women though this is quite rare.

As I said earlier, food is partly responsible for 30-40 percent (or even more) of all cancers.

These include but are not limited to lung cancer, colon cancer, bowel cancer, enlarged prostate, lung cancer, and of course, breast cancer.

Who Can Get Breast Cancer?

Being a woman is the biggest risk factor for breast cancer. As we've already seen, the female gender is the most affected group when it comes to breast cancer.

In fact, reports show that about 90 percent of all cases occur in women while the remaining 0.5 to 1 percent occur in men.

Other facts that can increase the risk of getting the disease include:

- Age (like I said earlier, women over 50 are usually at greater risk)
- Obesity or putting on more weight
- Having a family history of breast cancer
- Drinking too much (alcohol)
- Exposure to radiation
- Smoking or using tobacco harmfully
- Growing taller in adulthood
- Reproductive history (this includes issues like the age when you started having menstrual periods as well as when you had your first pregnancy)

Signs or Symptoms of Breast Cancer

Besides the risk factors, it's also important to be aware of some possible signs of breast cancer as this can help with early detection and diagnosis.

Here are the more common symptoms:

- Lump in the breast; you may also notice it underarm
- Nipple releasing a bloody discharge
- Changes in the texture or shape of the breast or nipple
- The breast may feel warmer; you may also notice swelling, redness, or darkening.
- Pulling of the breast
- Concentrated pain in a particular spot for long
- Itchiness of the nipple; may also develop a scaly sore or rash

While it's not all lumps that are connected to breast cancer, you should always check with a physician just to be sure, even if you don't experience any pain from the lump.

Getting a proper diagnosis, especially early, can greatly improve your chances of recovery.

Following a Plant-based Diet for Cancer Treatment

Several studies have shown that diet plays an important role in preventing most forms of cancer. Likewise, it can also contribute to your healing process after getting diagnosed. This is why you need to be more cautious of what you eat, especially after you've been diagnosed.

Generally, cancer patients are usually required to eat healthy in order to better cope physically and manage other symptoms as well as any side effects that may come with their treatment.

As a result, even when treating breast cancer medically, you may be required to follow a special diet with the aim that it will help to strengthen your immune system, help you cope with symptoms such as diarrhea and nausea, and provide additional nutrients such as protein.

Like I said earlier, even if you're not diagnosed, following the right diet will greatly lower your risk of developing the disease.

Generally, when it comes to breast cancer prevention, you want to follow a diet that is high in nuts and seeds, vegetables and mono-unsaturated fat (examples are olive oil and canola). The Dr. Barbara diet fulfills this criterion, which means it can serve as both a healing and maintenance diet.

Who is Barbara O'Neill and What is the Dr Barbara Diet?

Barbara O'Neill is the brain behind the Dr Barbara diet. If you're in the natural wellness space, you may have already heard about her.

Barbara is a health educator from Australia. She's also a nutritionist and naturopath and has several years of experience in the health industry.

As you may already know, her work is based on employing natural means to achieve optimal health and heal from diseases. Specifically, she believes in the power of food as medicine and advocates for plant-based nutrition.

The diet essentially focuses on eating whole foods from plant sources while limiting your intake of processed foods. These include foods such as nuts, seeds, fruits, vegetables, and legumes.

How the Dr. Barbara Diet Works

Dr Barbara believes that eating this way helps to balance the body's pH levels and maintains an alkaline environment which is necessary to heal from diseases such as breast cancer or prevent them in the first place.

So, to follow the Dr Barbara diet, you need to increase your intake of alkaline-forming foods (which are mostly plant-based) by at least 70 to 80 percent while reducing your consumption of acid-forming foods to not more than 20 percent.

Examples of alkaline-forming foods include certain fruits (which we will focus on in the recipe section), legumes, and dark leafy greens.

Examples of acid-forming foods include meat, sugar, dairy, and refined grains.

Best Foods for Breast Cancer Treatment and Prevention

As you can see, following a plant-based diet comes with a lot of benefits. However, when it comes to treating or preventing breast cancer, there are some foods that are generally better as they have anti-cancer properties.

With this in mind, here are 7 foods you should have in your pantry or list when dealing with cancer.

Fresh fruits

Examples include:

- Citrus fruits
- Ripe berries (particularly great if you have swallowing problems)
- Peaches
- Apples
- Pears
- Grapes

- Lime

- Tangerine

- Lemon

- Etc.

Nuts and seeds (great sources of Omega-3)

Examples include:

- Pecans

- Chia seeds

- Flaxseed

- Walnuts

- Almonds

- Brazil nuts

- Hazelnuts

- Pistachios

- Peanuts

Leafy greens

Examples include:

- Arugula

- Mustard greens

- Spinach

- Kale

- Watercress

- Cabbage

- Beets

- Etc.

Cruciferous vegetables (high in fiber and phytochemicals)

Examples include:

- Brussels sprouts

- Cauliflower

- Broccoli

- Cabbage

- Kale

- Bok choy

- Radish

- Rocket
- Turnips
- Wasabi
- Beans
- Etc.

Green tea (rich in antioxidants)

Drinking 2-3 cups of green tea a day can be very beneficial for cancer prevention and treatment.

Olive oil (a healthier option for your cooking needs)

Packed with polyphenols, oleuropein, and oleocanthal compounds which are all great at inhibiting cancer progression and providing anti-inflammatory benefits.

Herbs

Examples include:

- Oregano

- Onions

- Garlic

- Rosemary

- Turmeric

- Thyme

Worst Foods for Cancer

The chapter will be incomplete if you just go over the best foods and leave out those you should avoid. Thus, some of the worst foods for cancer are listed below:

- Refined carbs

- Processed meat

- Red meat

- Fried foods

- Fast foods

- Alcohol

- Refined sugar

- Ultra-processed foods

- Sugary foods and beverages

- Artificial sweeteners

You have to reduce your intake of these foods to the barest. Personally, I would recommend you completely avoid them!

Does Soy Cause Breast Cancer?

There are reports that suggest that soy products can increase the risk of developing breast cancer. The rationale behind this is that these products contain a high amount of isoflavones, which is linked to the development of breast cancer.

However, recent studies have proved this not to be accurate. In fact, on the contrary, reports show that increased soy intake could actually be associated with a lower risk of breast cancer. What's more, soy may also help to protect against recurrence in people who have already been diagnosed and treated.

Having said that, my personal recommendation is to eat a moderate amount of soy foods and not to go overboard. A moderate amount can be likened to 1 or 2 servings of whole soy foods like edamame and tofu every other day.

Other Helpful Lifestyle Considerations

- Try to maintain a moderate body weight

- Avoid certain skin care products, especially those that contain parabens. Instead, opt for natural skincare.

- Avoid exposure to pesticides and endocrine disruptors (like Bisphenol A)

- Engage in enough physical activities (get regular exercise)

- Avoid regular snacks; replace with whole, colorful fruits, which you can snack on between meals

- Try to sip 2-3 cups of green tea a day.

- Try to eat up to 2 ½ -3 cups of veggies and 1 ½ to 2 cups of fruits daily. Eat varieties!

- Opt for 100 percent whole grain foods such as cereals, bread, brown rice, millet, and quinoa.

- Quit smoking and drinking

Does Fasting Help With Breast Cancer?

Fasting is when you don't eat for a specific period of time. You may be wondering how this can be of any benefit to a cancer patient. Well, interestingly, fasting has proven to be significantly effective for shrinking cancer tumors and there's a lot of evidence to prove this, including testimonials from people who have battled cancer.

There are three main types of fasting - dry fasting, water fasting, and intermittent fasting.

Dry Fasting

Dry fasting simply means to go without food and water (as well as other fluids) for a specific period of time.

Water Fasting

Water fasting is when you skip food but drink water during the period of your fasting.

Intermittent Fasting

Intermittent fasting is simply following a time-restricted eating plan. In this case, each day, you eat at a specific time and fast during the rest of the time. The time you are eating is known as your eating window while the rest of the time is spent fasting or not eating.

How To Fast for Breast Cancer

A lot of people practice Intermittent fasting because it seems to be more convenient, especially if you're new to fasting.

As I said earlier, this type of fasting basically involves abstaining from food for a specific period of time during the day. For example, you may want to do a 16:8 hours intermittent fast; here you will fast for 16 hours and eat during the remaining 8 hours.

You are free to choose whatever time depending on your schedule but I've found it's easier to fast towards the night. So, you can have a fasting window of 6 pm on Monday to 12 noon on Tuesday, then eat between 12 noon to 6 pm.

You can repeat the cycle for as long as you want to depending on how many days you've set out to fast. It's recommended not to eat more than twice during your eating window and don't try to eat too much just to make up for the times you will not be eating. Eat your normal portion!

Personally, when fasting intermittently, I eat just once a day. This is known as OMAD - one meal a day.

Generally, I have found that a prolonged fast of up to 40 days or more helps with breast cancer healing.

Once you get comfortable fasting intermittently, you may want to try out water fasting. You may start with 3 days water fast. If water won't do, you can use juice. This is known as a juice fast. I have done a 14-day juice fast at one point in the past and the results were incredible.

Dr Barbara Alkaline Recipes for Breast Cancer

PECANS & BERRIES SALAD

Ingredients

- Baby arugula or mixed baby greens (15 oz pack)
- Blackberries (half pack, should weigh up to 3 oz)
- Raspberries (half pack, should weigh up to 3 oz)
- Fifteen pecan halves

To make the vinaigrette, here's what you need:

- 3 tbsp extra virgin olive oil
- ⅛ tsp kosher salt
- ⅛ tsp freshly ground pepper to taste
- 1 tbsp champagne vinegar (or rice vinegar/ apple cider vinegar)
- ½ tsp dried basil

Instructions

1. Let's start with the dressing/vinaigrette. Pour the vinegar into a bowl (make sure it's a bowl that won't react with the vinegar). Now add in the basil, pepper, and salt.

2. Next, you want to emulsify the olive oil with the vinaigrette. To do this, drizzle the oil in a slow stream; then whisk together until emulsified.

3. Now, combine the vinaigrette and baby arugula (or mixed greens) and transfer to a salad bowl.

4. Top with pecans, raspberries, and blackberries. Serve immediately.

BUTTERNUT SQUASH SOUP

Ingredients

- One tablespoon of olive oil
- One small onion, chopped

- Two tablespoons of fresh sage, chopped
- Six cups of butternut squash (peeled and cubed, should weigh about 30 oz)
- Half a teaspoon of kosher salt or sea salt
- One sweet apple (ideally, it should be large in size, you will need to peel and chop it)
- Half a teaspoon of cinnamon, grounded
- Half a teaspoon of paprika
- Four and a half cups of vegetable broth
- One tablespoon of fresh ginger, grated
- Half a cup of coconut milk (you can use more for garnish)
- ¼ tsp fresh nutmeg, grated

Instructions

1. Start by preheating your oven to 400 degrees F. Next, mix the apple, sage, squash, cinnamon, onion, paprika, and ¼ tsp salt in a Dutch oven. Toss in one tablespoon of olive oil and combine very well.
2. Roast until the squash becomes tender. This usually takes about half an hour.

3. After that, transfer the Dutch oven to the stove and add in the coconut milk, broth, nutmeg, ginger, and ¼ tsp salt. Allow to boil.

4. Next, you want to blend the mixture. You can either use an immersion blender or you can transfer the soup to the blender in batches. Blend until you get a smooth consistency.

5. When serving, you can drizzle extra coconut milk on top and if you like, add a pinch of nutmeg.

CARROT BANANA PROTEIN DRINK

Ingredients

- ¼ cup unflavored pea protein powder (you can substitute this with whey protein)
- Half a teaspoon of turmeric
- One cup of almond milk
- One medium-sized banana, riped
- Two baby carrots
- One tablespoon of ground flax

- Agave syrup (or any other natural sweetener of your choice)
- Ice

Instructions

1. Add all the ingredients to a blender and blend until you get a smooth consistency. Enjoy!

SUPERFOOD SMOOTHIE

Ingredients

- 1 date, pitted
- Half medium-sized banana, riped
- Half a tablespoon of chia seeds
- One tablespoon of raw shelled hemp seeds (you can substitute this with any other seed of your choice)
- ¾ cup of baby kale or spinach
- ¾ cup unsweetened vanilla almond milk

- One cup of ice

Instructions

1. Add everything to a blender or high-speed food processor and blend until you get a smooth consistency. Enjoy!

LEMON BRUSSEL SPROUTS

Ingredients

- ¼ cup fresh lemon juice
- Half a cup of chicken broth or low-sodium vegetable broth
- Zest from one lemon
- Two pounds of Brussel sprouts, the ends should be trimmed
- Two teaspoons of kosher salt
- ¼ teaspoon of fresh ground pepper

Instructions

1. Start by shredding the sprouts; you can do this with the slicing disk on a food processor or a sharp knife. If you're using a sharp knife, you will need to halve the sprouts before thinly slicing by hand.

2. Pour the broth into a deep skillet and heat over medium heat. Once it begins to simmer, add in the shredded sprouts and season with the pepper and salt.

3. Sauté and stir frequently until the sprouts become a little wilted. This should take about 8-10 minutes. Then remove the skillet from heat.

4. You can stir in the lemon zest and juice if you plan to serve right away, otherwise stir in the lemon just before you serve it hot or warm anytime.

CHOCOLATE BANANA DRINK

Ingredients

- Six ounces of carob-flavored soy milk (can be substituted with fortified cocoa)
- One banana, diced and frozen
- One pinch of cinnamon

Instructions

1. Combine everything in a blender and blend until smooth. Serve immediately.

KIWIFRUIT SHAKE

Ingredients

- 4 cups non-fat vanilla vegan yogurt, frozen
- 2 sliced kiwifruit

Instructions

1. Add both ingredients to a blender or food processor
   and blend until smooth. Serve.

LEMON QUINOA SALAD

Ingredients

- One cup of lentils, cooked
- One cup of quinoa, cooked
- Three tablespoons of olive oil
- One minced garlic clove
- Half a cup of yellow bell pepper, chopped
- Half a cup of red bell pepper, chopped
- ¼ cup freshly squeezed lemon juice
- ¼ cup red onion, chopped
- Salt to taste

Instructions

1. Combine all the ingredients (except salt) in a large bowl. Season with salt to taste.

2. You can season with more grounded pepper if you wish. Serve.

ELECTRIC SALAD

Ingredients

- 1 cup cherry tomatoes
- 2 red onions
- 1 handful romaine lettuce
- 1 lime (you will need the juice)
- 1 cup kale, chopped
- 3 jalapenos
- Olive oil
- 1 yellow pepper
- 1 orange pepper

Instructions

1. The first thing is to wash and rinse all the ingredients if you have not already done so. Once dry, cut them into smaller pieces.
2. Combine everything in a bowl and drizzle with the lemon juice and oil. Enjoy!

QUINOA PORRIDGE

Ingredients

- ½ tsp cayenne
- ½ lime (you will need to grate the skin)
- 1 cup dry quinoa
- 2 cups water
- ½ cup coconut milk (can be substituted with cream if you wish)
- Cloves to taste

- ½ handful assorted nuts and seeds (optional)

Instructions

1. Prepare the quinoa according to the instructions on the package.
2. After that, pour it into a saucepan (this should be after you have drained the quinoa). Then add the cloves and cayenne. Stir well to combine.
3. Next, add the milk and grated lime (you can also add grated apple if you wish). Stir well to mix.
4. Top with nuts and seeds. Enjoy!

ALKALINE MILLET

Ingredients

- ½ tsp sea salt
- 2 ½ cup water

- 1 cup millet

Instructions

1. The first thing is to dry sauté the millet until golden brown. Then add in the water and salt.
2. Bring the mixture to a boil, then simmer until the water is absorbed. This usually takes about 30 minutes but it could be more depending on the heat.
3. Let everything cool with the lid on. Serve and enjoy!

ZUCCHINI AND HEART MUSHROOM SOUP

Ingredients

- 1 medium zucchini, chopped
- 1 medium-sized onion, chopped (if you eat onion a lot, then you can use a large onion instead)
- 2 bay leaves
- Any vegetable stock of your choice (ideally, homemade)

- 1 tsp grapeseed oil

- 1 lb mushroom, mixed and chopped

- Cayenne pepper to taste

- Sea salt to taste

- Sweet basil to taste

Instructions

1. Start by setting your stove to medium heat. Set a pan with a heavy base on top of the stove, then add the grapeseed oil. Once it gets a little hot, add in the onion and sauté for 5 minutes.

2. Next, add the mushrooms, basil, and bay leaves. Allow it to cook for an additional five minutes, then add the zucchini. Cook until the vegetables release their juices. This might take up to 10-15 minutes.

3. Now, pour in the vegetable stock and bring to a boil. Then reduce the heat and simmer for five minutes.

4. Finally, remove the bay leaves from the soup before seasoning with salt and pepper. Serve!

MUSHROOM & ONION GRAVY

Ingredients

- 2-3 cups of spring water
- ½ cup mushroom
- 1 tsp sea salt
- ½ cup onion
- ½ tsp oregano
- ¼ cup cayenne
- ½ tsp thyme
- 2 tbsp grapeseed oil
- 3 tbsp garbanzo bean flour
- 1 tsp onion powder

Instructions

1. Start by pouring the grapeseed oil into your frying pan. Then set it on the stove over medium or high heat.
2. Once the oil is a bit hot, add the onion and mushroom and sauté for a minute. Then add the other seasonings and spices, except the cayenne.

3. Sauté for five minutes, then add 2 cups of spring water and the cayenne. Stir well to mix and allow to boil.

4. While you're waiting, sift in the flour little by little, then use a whisk to stir it well in order to reduce lumps.

5. Continue cooking until it boils. You can add more water if you want but don't add not more than one cup. Serve.

GINGER TEA

Ingredients

- 1 pinch cayenne
- 1 thumb fresh ginger root (can be substituted with the powder)
- 4 cups spring water
- 2 tbsp fresh lime juice
- 2 sprigs of new organic dill weed
- Raw agave to taste

Instructions

1. Start by boiling the spring water.

2. While you're waiting, peel the ginger root, then chop
   it into tiny pieces and add to the boiling water. Also,
   add the weed.

3. Let it cook for 5 minutes, then strain the tea into a
   glass jar. Add the lime juice and cayenne and stir.

4. Finally, add the agave to taste. You can have it either
   hot or cold.

AVOCADO BOWL

Ingredients

- Fresh lime juice from 1 lime
- ½ cup cucumber, chopped
- 2 tbsp melted coconut oil
- 16-20 basil leaves (can be substituted with parsley
  leaves)

- 1 avocado

- Nuts, chopped

- ⅛ tsp lime zest (you can use more for serving)

- 1 pinch salt

- Agave to taste (optional)

Instructions

1. Start by pouring the lime juice into a blender. Add the avocado and agave. Then blend the mixture until smooth.

2. Now, add the lime zest, cucumber, salt, and coconut oil. Blend again until smooth.

3. Then add the basil or parsley leaves and mix a bit.

4. Transfer to a bowl and top with the chopped nuts. You can top with more lime zest if desired.

FRUIT SALAD

Ingredients

- One pint of fresh blueberries
- One ripe pear, cored and diced
- One pint of fresh strawberries, sliced (no stems)
- Two cups grapes, deseeded
- 2 tbsp date syrup (optional)
- ¼ tsp ground cinnamon
- 2 tbsp freshly squeezed lemon juice

Instructions

1. Combine all the ingredients in a bowl. Store in a refrigerator. Serve chill.

HERBERT HUMMUS

Ingredients

- Two garlic cloves

- One cup of fresh basil leaves, blanched and lightly packed
- Four cups of cooked garbanzo beans
- Juice from one lemon
- One cup of vegetable broth
- Half a cup of tarragon leaves, blanched and lightly packed
- Half a cup of fresh, flat parsley leaves
- ¼ cup of chives, chopped
- 2 tbsp sesame seeds, toasted

Instructions

1. Start by dabbing the basil leaves and tarragon until they dry. Now, cut them into smaller bits and put in a blender or food processor.
2. Add in the beans, sesame seeds, lemon juice, garlic, and vegetable broth. Blend until smooth and creamy. Add the chives; stir and serve.

NB: Consume within 4 days.

MISO NOODLE SOUP

Ingredients

- Two scallions, sliced
- One cup of adzuki beans (cooked or canned)
- Four tablespoons of miso
- Two tablespoons of fresh cilantro/basil, chopped
- Seven ounces of soba noodles (100% buckwheat)
- Four cups of water

Instructions

1. Start by pouring some water into a large pot; bring it to a boil.
2. Next, add in the soba noodles and stir. Cook for about five minutes, then drain and rinse (use hot water).
3. In another pot, pour in some water and bring to boil. Remove from heat and add in the miso and stir until dissolved.

4. Finally, add the noodles, adzuki beans, scallions and cilantro to the miso broth. Stir well to combine. Serve warm.

HEMP MILK

Ingredients

- Spring water
- 6 tbsp sea moss gel
- 1 cup hemp seeds

Instructions

1. Start by soaking the hemp seeds in 6 cups of spring water for 30 minutes.
2. Next, transfer the seeds with the water into a blender and blend until smooth.
3. Add in the sea moss and blend for 30 seconds. Store in the refrigerator and use within four days.

TASTY PANINI

Ingredients

- 1 tsp cinnamon
- ¼ cup natural peanut butter
- ¼ cup raisin
- ¼ cup hot water
- Whole grain bread, 2 slices
- 1 ripe banana, peeled and chopped
- 2 tsp cacao powder

Instructions

1. Start by pouring the hot water into a bowl. Add the cinnamon, raisin, and cacao powder and combine.
2. Next, spread the peanut butter on each of the bread slices.
3. Place the chopped banana on the toast.

4. Next, transfer the raisin mixture into a blender and blend until smooth. Spread on the sandwich. Enjoy!

BASIC POLENTA

Ingredients

- One and a half cups of coarse cornmeal
- Five cups of water
- ¾ tsp salt

Instructions

1. Start by pouring the water into a saucepan. Put it on a stove and set to low heat.
2. Gradually add the cornmeal into the water. Then stir until creamy. This might take a couple of minutes.
3. Season with the salt, then transfer the polenta into a bowl. Refrigerate for an hour, then serve.

KALE SALAD & HEMP RANCH

Ingredients

- One teaspoon of dill

- Half a teaspoon of sea salt

- Half a cup of hemp seeds

- Two tablespoons of squeezed lime juice

- Half butternut squash, cubed

- Six cups of chopped kale

- Two teaspoons of salt

- One to two tablespoons of grapeseed oil

Instructions

1. Switch on the oven and heat it to up to 350-400 degrees F.

2. Put the hemp seeds, dill, and lime juice in a blender and blend until smooth. You can also use a food processor.

3. Now, toss the kale and squash in the grapeseed oil and add the sea salt. Transfer to a baking dish and roast for 15 to 20 minutes or until cooked. You will know this when the kale gets crispy.

4. Allow to cook, then you can top with dressings.

AVOCADO LETTUCE WRAPS

Ingredients

- One teaspoon of sea salt
- Two avocados, sliced
- One teaspoon of fresh lime juice
- Twelve romaine lettuce leaves
- Two diced bell peppers
- Half red onion (should be diced and sliced)
- Three plum tomatoes, chopped

- One to two teaspoons of cayenne pepper

Instructions

1. Mix all the ingredients in a bowl except the romaine lettuce.
2. Next, you want to wash the lettuce separately. Allow it to dry.
3. Now, place the dry leaves on a plate or dish in such a way that each one forms a natural scoop.
4. Next, pour the mixture you prepared from step one into each leaf so that it fills it. Now, you have your avocado lettuce wraps. Enjoy!

RYE TOMATO & AVOCADO SANDWICH

Ingredients

- Two slices of rye bread
- Two sliced plum tomatoes

- One avocado, sliced

- One to two teaspoons of sea salt

- One to three tablespoons of olive oil

- Half a cup of dandelion greens or purslane

Instructions

1. Place the avocado slices on top of the bread slices.

2. Next, drizzle with olive oil. It should go on top of the avocado.

3. Now, arrange the tomato slices on top of the avocados. You can sprinkle some salt if you wish.

4. Finally, top with purslane. Enjoy your sandwich.

GRANOLA PLATE

Things You Need

- Two and a half cups of oats

- A cup of shredded coconut, unsweetened without preservatives
- 1 tsp of vanilla, extract
- ¾ cup of almonds
- ¼ cup of maple syrup (should be pure)
- ¼ cup of pumpkin seeds
- ½ cup of walnuts (only use if you tolerate it)
- ¼ tsp cinnamon (optional)
- ⅛ tsp of sea salt
- 2 tbsp of coconut oil
- Dried mango to taste (optional, must come without any preservatives)

Cooking Instructions

1. Start by preheating your oven. Set the temperature at 300 degrees Fahrenheit.
2. Transfer the almonds, oats, and walnuts onto cookie sheet.
3. Next, get a small pot and mix the other ingredients - coconut oil, syrup, cinnamon, salt and vanilla. Now pour the mixture on top of the oats and walnuts and flip to mix it up.

4. Then bake for 18-22 minutes. Make sure to stir every 8-10 minutes.

5. When you're done, take it out of the oven, then add the pumpkin seeds and coconut.

6. Bake for an extra 10 to 15 minutes, then take it out and move to a Pyrex dish to get it to cool. Once again, you want to stir often.

7. Optionally, you can cut the dried mango into tiny slices and mix with the granola. Otherwise, skip this step if it's not tolerated. Put it in the fridge to cool.

"MINT" ICED TEA

Things You Need

- 1 tbsp of mint leaves (fresh, ideally should come in a sachet or tea ball)
- Chamomile tea (a bag should be enough)
- 1 teaspoon of sweetener (agave syrup/you can also use raw honey though this is not permitted in Dr Barbara's guide)

Cooking Instructions

1. Get a medium-sized teapot and fill it with water.
    Now, soak (or steep) the tea for 18-20 minutes.

2. Remove the mint and chamomile. Add your
    preferred sweetener and stir well. Allow it to cool
    down, then put it in the fridge.

WATERMELON SALAD

Things You Need

- One red watermelon (small or half-size, seedless)
- One to two cups of English cucumber (sliced)
- Mint sprigs to taste (make sure it's fresh)
- ***Blueberries (one half-pint box)***

Cooking Instructions

1. Slice the watermelon into tiny pieces. Next, "scrape off" the outer part, then cut into very small chunks.

2. Transfer the chunks to 1 large bowl or you can divide it into smaller bowls.

3. Next, add the cucumber slices and use the blueberries and sprigs as toppings.

Zucchini & Plum Tomatoes

Ingredients

- Half a tablespoon of Herbes de Provence (you can find how to make this online)
- One medium-sized zucchini (cut into bits)
- Five medium-sized fresh plum tomatoes, diced
- Two tablespoons of extra virgin olive oil
- Five garlic cloves, smashed
- Fresh pepper and kosher salt to taste

Instructions

1. Pour the olive oil into a large non-stick skillet and heat. Set the stove to medium-high heat.

2. Add in the garlic and sauté until it turns golden. This should take about a minute or two.

3. Now, add in salt and pepper followed by zucchini.

4. Leave it to cook for 4 to 5 minutes on each side. Then introduce the plum tomatoes and Herbes de Provence. You can add additional salt if you desire.

5. Reduce the heat and simmer for 5 to 10 minutes. Serve.

Baked Bananas

Ingredients

- 1 banana (ideally, it should be medium ripped; cut it into half lengthwise)
- Half a tablespoon of honey
- Cinnamon to taste

Instructions

1. Start by preheating the oven to 400 degrees F.

2. Arrange the banana halves on a foil or oven-safe dish. Sprinkle with honey and cinnamon.

3. Cover tight with foil, then place it in the oven and allow to bake for 10-15 minutes. Enjoy!

4. Optionally, you can serve with light ice cream or whipped cream.

Conclusion

Most breast cancer patients are often required to follow a specific diet to ensure healthy eating and aid their recovery. Some women may also do the same to reduce the risk of getting the disease or prevent a recurrence.

Regardless of where you stand, you will greatly benefit from following the Dr Barbara diet.

While it can be strict for many people as it focuses mainly on foods from plant sources, it gets easier with time. In this book, I have talked about the importance of fasting as a great complement to the Dr Barbara diet as I believe this is one of the best ways to facilitate healing from breast cancer naturally.